CW01474905

Practical Remedies with Doctor Cip

Ciprian Nicolae and Delia Nicolae

Published by Ciprian Nicolae, 2023.

PRACTICAL REMEDIES WITH DOCTOR CIP

First edition. February 21, 2023.

Copyright © 2023 Ciprian Nicolae and Delia Nicolae.

ISBN: 979-8215408148

Written by Ciprian Nicolae and Delia Nicolae.

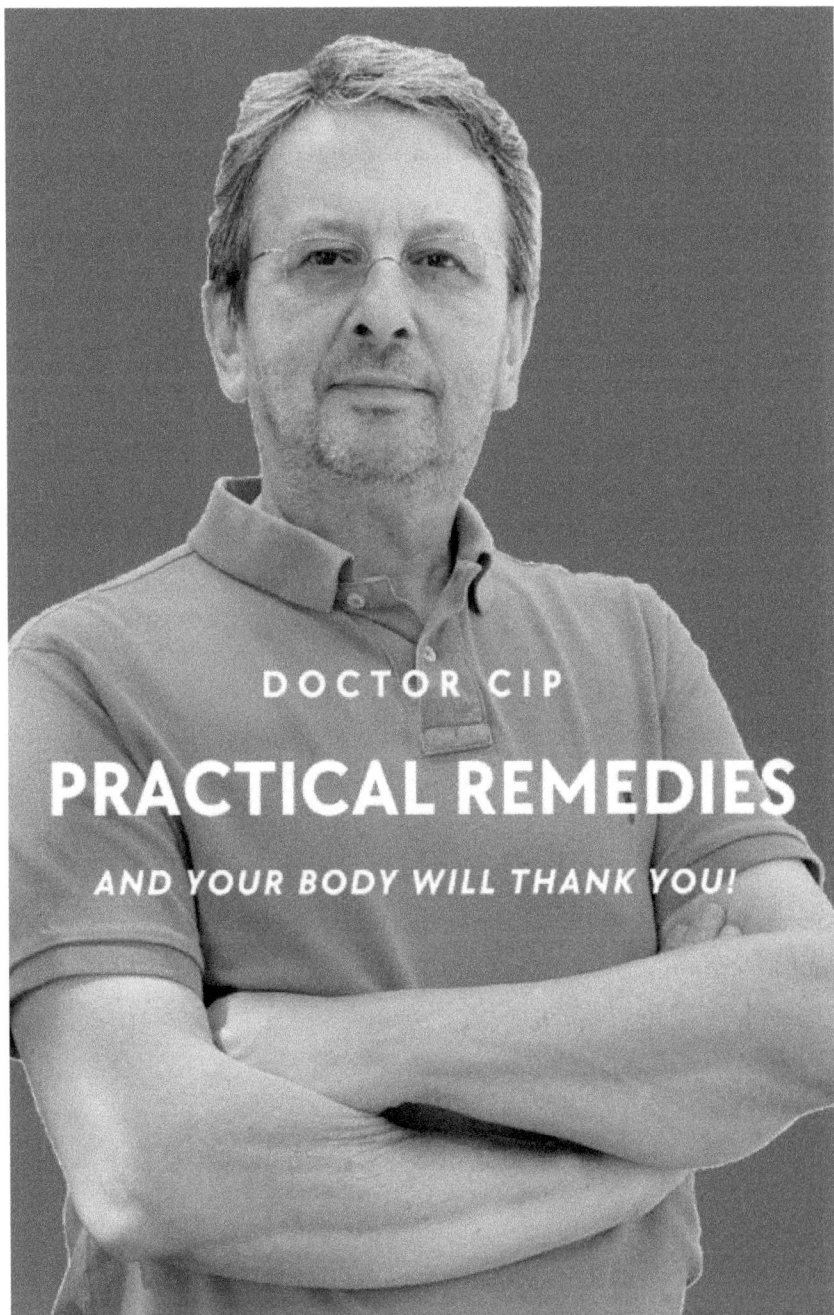

DOCTOR CIP

PRACTICAL REMEDIES

AND YOUR BODY WILL THANK YOU!

CIPRIAN NICOLAE
Paintings
Delia Nicolae

PRACTICAL REMEDIES
WITH
DOCTOR CIP

And your body will thank you!

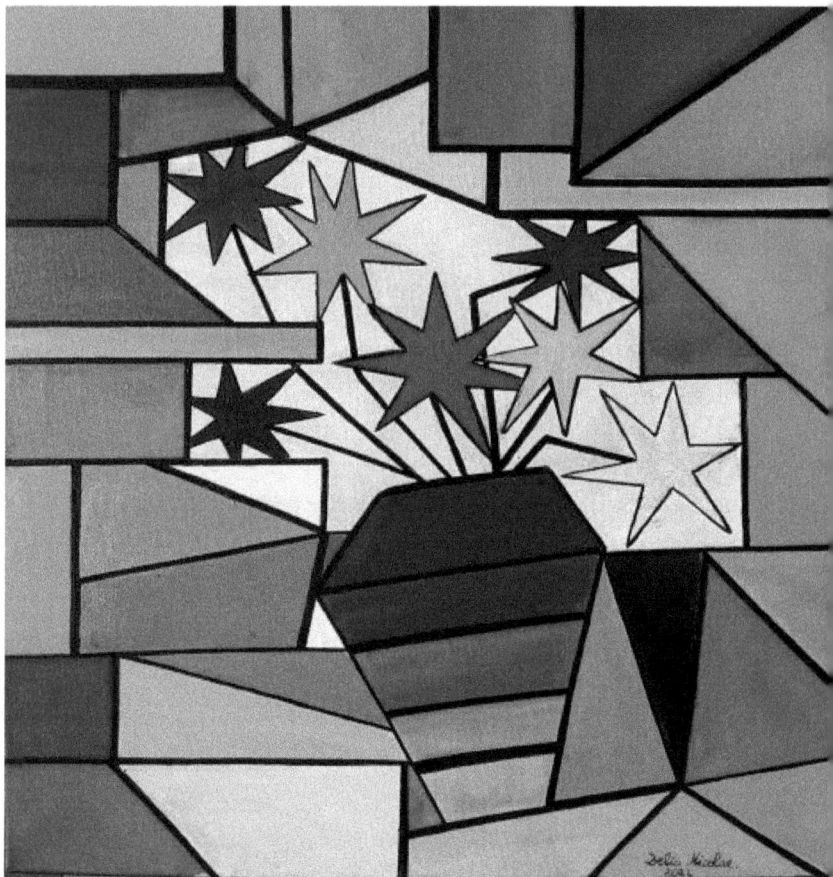

INTRODUCTION

In this book I present practical remedies for common ailments.

These remedies do not replace the visit to the doctor or the possible treatments indicated by him, but complement them.

I have collected them over time from different sources, and presented them many times in videos on social platforms and following the many requests I received in this regard, I decided to collect them in this volume.

So, apply these remedies and your body will thank you for it!

RESPIRATORY DISEASES

In this chapter I present some solutions for the situation in which you have persistent cough and mucus, some maneuvers for cleaning the airways and simple but very effective solutions for preventing and treating colds.

I will also present some useful measures in bronchial asthma and Chronic Obstructive Pulmonary Disease (COPD).

Cough and persistent mucus

Honey and lemon solution for coughs and sore throats

Ingredients

1. Two spoons of honey.
2. Two lemons, preferably with untreated peel. If they are treated, you have two possibilities:

- you only use the juice.

- you leave them for 15 minutes in 500 ml of warm water in which you put a spoonful of baking soda, wash them with this solution and then rinse them under running water. In this way, most of the chemical substances with which they were treated are removed and you can use the whole lemons, including the peel.

3. 500 ml of water.

Preparation method

Put the water, the two spoons of honey, the two sliced lemons (or just the juice) in the blender and mix well.

The solution is kept in the refrigerator and you drink it throughout the day with small sips.

Solution with brown sugar, bay leaves and lemon for coughs and sore throats

Ingredients

1. Brown sugar
2. Water
3. Bay leaves
4. Lemons, preferably with untreated peel: only the juice is used from one lemon, and the second lemon is cut into slices, if it is untreated, and if it is treated, you have two possibilities:

- you only use the juice.

- you leave it for 15 minutes in 500 ml of warm water in which you put a spoonful of baking soda, then you wash it with this solution and finally, you rinse it under running water.

Preparation method

● Put 12 spoons of brown sugar in a pot, which is put on the stove, on low heat, until the sugar melts;

● Add 400 ml of water;

● When the water starts to boil and the sugar has dissolved, add 10 bay leaves and let it boil for 15 minutes;

● When the syrup cools down, strain it and add the lemon juice and slices;

● Keep in the refrigerator and take 3 tablespoons a day.

Remedies for persistent mucus

There are many people who have mucus in their throats for months or years, an unpleasant situation both for these people and for those around them, due to the constant need to clear the throat.

These people try all kinds of treatments, but the situation does not improve.

The causes are multiple: gastroesophageal reflux, allergies, infections, asthma, smoking, chronic bronchitis.

Remedies

1. consume very hot liquids: tea, soup, water, which have a mucolytic effect (liquefies the mucus), which is thus eliminated;

2. do inhalations with boiling water in which you put eucalyptol and/or menthol;

3. gargle with salt water: a spoonful of salt dissolved in a glass of water;

4. if you have no contraindications, take 1-2 teaspoons of honey daily, which, in addition to its antibacterial and antiviral properties, also has a mucolytic effect (liquefies the mucus), favoring its elimination;

5. very good mucolytic effect also has chili, added to drink or food;

6. put a drop of oregano oil under the tongue, with very good effects;

7. thyme capsules or dried thyme leaves: dilates the bronchioles and liquefies the mucus;

8. very important: drink at least 2-2.5 l of liquids daily;

9. rest well, sleep for 8 hours, on your back, with your head on a large pillow, so that the mucus does not reach the throat.

Cleaning the respiratory tract

The state of the lungs is very important, because all metabolic processes in the body depend on the amount of oxygen in the blood, so the measures we can take to ensure that we have the cleanest lungs are welcome.

These methods are especially recommended for smokers and those who have quit smoking.

Postural drainage exercises

In all exercises, inhale slowly through the nose and exhale slowly through the mouth, making sure that the exhalation is 2 times longer than the inhalation (for example: you breathe in for 4 seconds and exhale it in 8 seconds).

First exercise: lie on the floor with a pillow under your head and 2-3 pillows under your knees, keeping your legs bent. Breathe in this position for a few minutes.

The second exercise: lie on your side with a pillow or hand under your head and a pillow under your hip.

Breathe in this position for a few minutes.

Repeat the exercise turned on the other side.

The third exercise: lie on your stomach with 2-3 pillows under it, so that your bottom is above your legs and head.

The hands are bent and kept under the floor, resting the head on them.

Breathe in this position for a few minutes.

Repeat the exercises 4-5 times a week.

Through these exercises, secretions from the lungs reach the upper respiratory tract and are eliminated through coughing.

ATTENTION: do not do these exercises for 2 hours after eating.

They are best done in the morning or in the evening, before going to bed.

Dry cough

Many times, the dry, persistent cough is caused by a contraction of the muscles of the larynx, determined by the irritation caused by a virus.

A very simple and effective remedy is the administration of lactic calcium for a week, in a dose of 2 tablets 3 times a day for adults, and for children, 1 tablet 3 times a day.

Cold

If you have a cold, stuffy nose, sore throat, cough with expectoration, you can apply the following remedies:

Salt water gargle

Put 2-3 tablespoons of salt in a liter of warm water, mix well to dissolve the salt and then gargle with this solution.

Salt water inhalations

Put 2 liters of water on the stove, add 3-4 tablespoons of salt and when the water starts to boil, turn off the heat and inhale the steam.

Salt has an antibacterial, antiviral, anti-inflammatory effect, it liquefies secretions, which are thus easily eliminated.

Solution with honey, apple cider vinegar, lemon and turmeric

In 500 ml of water, put 2 spoons of honey (careful, it should not be adulterated), 2 spoons of apple cider vinegar, the juice of a lemon or a lemon cut into pieces, if it has untreated peel, 1 spoon of turmeric (curcuma), 2 tablespoons of extra virgin olive oil and 1 teaspoon of ground pepper and mix well in a blender. Keep the mixture in the refrigerator and take 50 ml 3-4 times a day.

Note: Olive oil and ground pepper are added to increase the absorption of turmeric.

Cardamom

Put half a teaspoon of cardamom (this is a spice) in 100 ml of warm water and drink this solution 3 times a day.

Thyme

Take half a teaspoon of dry thyme 2-3 times a day, which has an antibacterial and secretion-fluidizing effect.

Oregano

Take 2-3 times a day oregano oil (liquid or capsules), which has an antibacterial, antiviral and anti-inflammatory effect.

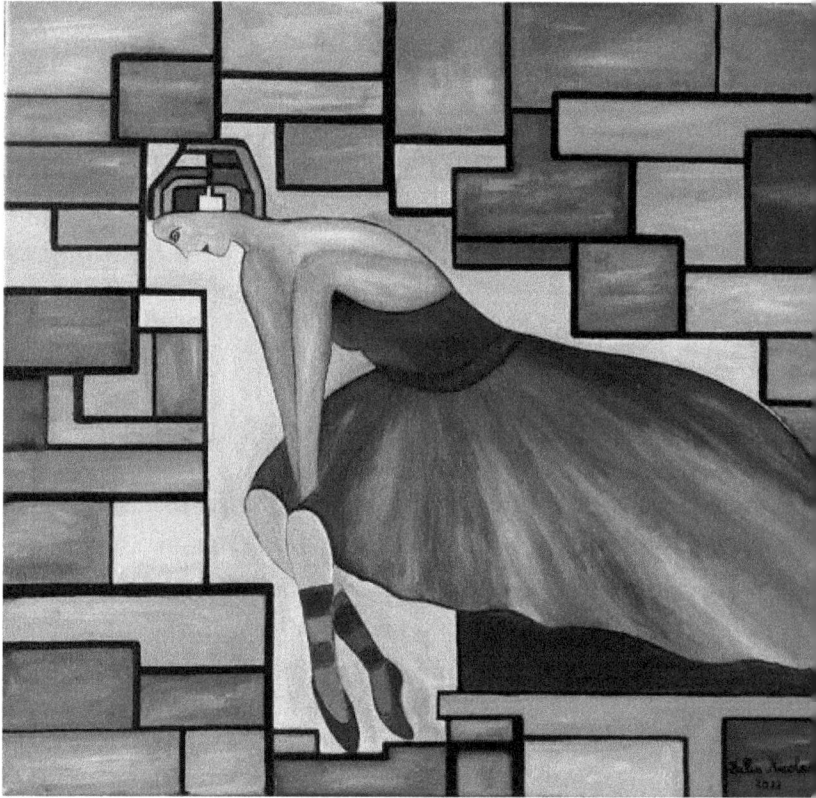

Bronchial asthma

Bronchial asthma is characterized by the obstruction of the small airways, so that, during the crisis, the person cannot expel the air from the lungs.

Most of the time, the cause is allergic in nature, that is, the body secretes excess antibodies against certain substances, which are called allergens.

I found very interesting information about the treatment of asthma, namely that vitamin D relieves asthma, in the sense that it reduces the frequency and intensity of attacks. So, it is not about the treatment of the crisis, which is an emergency treatment, which aims to resume normal breathing.

The long-term treatment of asthma has two goals:

1. reducing the allergic reaction, which is an exaggerated immune reaction. For this purpose, cortisone drugs are frequently used, which have the effect of reducing immunity, but which, especially in long-term use, have serious adverse effects. Vitamin D has the effect of regulating immunity, without, however, having the adverse effects of cortisones;

2. reducing the inflammation that occurs in the small airways. For this purpose, cortisones are also frequently used, which have an anti-inflammatory effect, but which, as I said, especially in long-term use, have serious adverse effects. Vitamin D has an anti-inflammatory effect, without, however, having the adverse effects of cortisones.

In addition, vitamin D also has the effect of increasing the sensitivity of cellular receptors for cortisol, so that the necessary dose of corticosteroids decreases, which also leads to the reduction of their adverse effects.

Vitamin D3 can be administered in a dose of 20,000 iu per day, associated with vitamin K2, 200 micrograms per day and magnesium, 500 mg per day.

For better absorption, it is recommended that vitamin D3 be taken with a meal or with a spoonful of olive oil.

Note: vitamin K2 is not involved in clotting, it is different from vitamin K1 (or vitamin K as it is commonly called), which has a role in clotting and is available only by prescription. Vitamin K2 is released without a prescription!

Chronic sinusitis

If you have chronic sinusitis, the following two remedies can be helpful:

1. nasal irrigation with a solution of xylitol and grapefruit seed extract. There is a commercial preparation that contains these two ingredients, which I found here: https://xlear.ro/xlear-neti-rinse-irigator-pentru-ingrijirea-sinusurilor (no, I'm not advertising, I have nothing to do with the company).

You can also prepare it yourself, from xylitol and grapefruit seed extract.

Xylitol has an effect of inhibiting the formation of biofilm, which is formed by calcium deposits on the sinus mucosa, deposits in which bacteria "hide".

Grapefruit seed extract has antibacterial and antifungal action.

You wash your nose twice a day for a week.

2. nasal irrigation with a garlic infusion, which is prepared as follows: cut two cloves of garlic into small pieces, put them in a cheesecloth or colander, which you immerse in hot water, wait for the water to become lukewarm , strain the solution (make sure no piece of garlic remains), put it in an irrigator and do nasal washes 2-3 times a day, for a week.

COPD

COPD is a condition characterized by a narrowing of the small airways.

The cause is represented in most cases by smoking. At the level of the alveoli and bronchioles, inflammation and oxidative processes occur, the consequence of which is the difficulty of gas exchange, with the reduction of the amount of oxygen that enters the blood and the amount of CO2 that passes from the blood into the exhaled air. Over time, these inflammatory lesions lead to the replacement of normal tissues with fibrous tissue, resulting in pulmonary fibrosis, which causes a reduction in lung elasticity and increasingly difficult breathing.

The disease is considered irreversible, although the latest studies show that there may be a certain degree of reversibility.

In any case, the treatment must have two goals:

1. reduction of inflammation and oxidative processes, to stop the evolution of the disease;

2. reducing the amount of exhaled CO2, so that the respiratory effort decreases and the patient's comfort improves.

Thus, the following measures must be taken:

1. stopping smoking, which is **mandatory**!

2. diet without or with a massive reduction in carbohydrates (sugar, flour, potatoes, rice) and switching to a predominantly meat-based diet. Thus, the amount of carbon dioxide (CO2) produced in the body decreases significantly and since there is less CO2 to exhale, the effort to exhale is automatically reduced, and the patient's comfort increases;

3. intermittent fasting, which has several beneficial effects, which add up: strong anti-inflammatory effect, the triggering of autophagy, through which abnormal proteins are recycled into normal proteins (thus, it is possible that part of the fibrous tissue is reduced).

I have read many reports of patients who achieved significant improvements with no carb and intermittent fasting alone.

4. vitamin D3, up to 40,000 iu per day, associated with vitamin K2, 400 micrograms and magnesium, 500 mg. Vitamin D has a strong anti-inflammatory effect, similar to cortisone, without, however, having its adverse effects;

Note: vitamin K2 is not involved in clotting, it is different from vitamin K1 (or vitamin K as it is commonly called), which has a role in clotting and is available only by prescription. Vitamin K2 is released without a prescription!

5. vitamin E, in the form of tocotrienols, which is much stronger than the form of tocopherols. Vitamin E has a powerful antioxidant and fibrous tissue reduction effect. The dose is 300 mg x 3 times a day;

6. natural vitamin C, not synthetic: it has an anti-inflammatory, antioxidant effect and studies show that it increases alveolar respiratory exchange;

8. melatonin: 3 mg per day, which has a strong antioxidant effect, thus improving breathing.

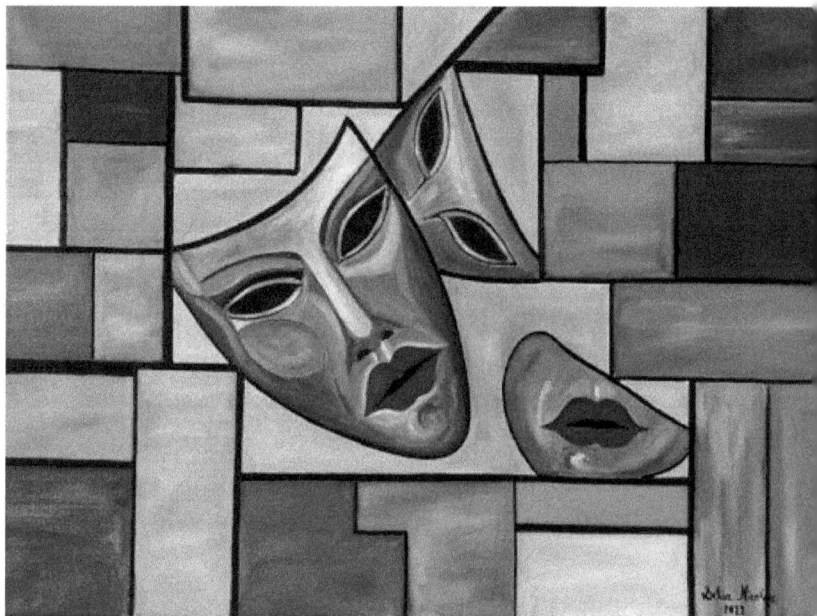

DIGESTIVE DISEASES

In this chapter I will present remedies for a series of digestive ailments or symptoms.

Gastroesophageal reflux

Gastroesophageal reflux is manifested by a burning sensation in the chest, which generally occurs after a meal or during the night.

Although many people believe that gastroesophageal reflux is caused by an increase in gastric acidity, it is actually caused, in most cases, by a decrease in it.

The explanation is as follows: the muscle that closes and opens the opening between the esophagus and the stomach is stimulated by the increase in gastric acidity, which occurs during digestion, to prevent food from returning to the esophagus from the stomach. When gastric acidity decreases, the muscle is weakly stimulated, and the orifice closes insufficiently, so that the gastric juice flows back into the esophagus. Although its acidity is low, it is, however, too high for the esophageal mucosa, which is not built to withstand acidic substances, not even slightly acidic ones.

As such, the remedy is represented by increasing gastric acidity, by administering betaine hydrochloride at the beginning of the meal. It starts with 2 capsules and depending on the results, it can be increased up to 4-6 capsules. The treatment is continued for a month, then it can be stopped, because, in most cases, gastric acidity returns to normal.

If the reflux occurs during sleep, it is recommended to put a 2-3 cm thick board under the mattress, at the level of the head, so that the esophagus is slightly above the stomach, so that the gastric juice does not flow back into the esophagus.

Bloating

The five most common causes of bloating are:

Decreased gastric acidity, situation in which bloating is accompanied by gastro-oesophageal reflux (burning on the chest). Protein digestion takes place in the stomach, and for this it is necessary that the gastric acidity is high. If the acidity decreases, the proteins are not fully digested, so that the undigested proteins end up in the colon, where they undergo a process of putrefaction, with the release of gases, which cause bloating.

(For treatment, see section about gastroesophageal reflux.)

Decrease in the amount of bile, which occurs in the case of gallstones (gallstones) or lazy gallbladder. Bile is necessary for the digestion of fats, so when there is not enough bile, the fats are not digested completely, they end up undigested in the colon, where they undergo a putrefaction process, with the release of gas and a feeling of bloating.

In this case, bloating is accompanied by constipation and pain under the right rib, which can radiate to the neck.

Treatment consists of administration of purified bile salts (eg "amrase" or "bile acid factors Jarrow").

Deficiency of pancreatic enzymes: in this case, bloating is accompanied by diarrhea and stool with a greasy appearance. Treatment is the administration of pancreatic enzymes (eg, triferment).

SIBO syndrome, which is an excess of bacteria in the small intestine, where normally very few microbes are found. Under their influence, food ferments and gases are produced. The treatment is represented by a diet without dietary fiber (fruits, vegetables) and without fermented foods (kefir, pickles, sauerkraut) for one month and the administration of essential oil of oregano, garlic capsules or essential oil of cloves, which destroy excess bacteria.

Attention: essential oils are diluted, not taken as such. You can dissolve 2 drops in a tablespoon of olive or coconut oil, mixing well.

The imbalance of the microbial flora from the colon (large intestine), a situation produced by a low consumption of dietary fiber. The treatment is represented by the consumption of vegetables and fruits, which have fiber, fermented foods (kefir, pickles), which contain bacteria and the administration of probiotics. All these measures contribute to restoring the microbial balance in the colon.

Irritable colon

Irritable bowel syndrome is manifested by abdominal discomfort, pain, bloating, diarrhea and/or constipation.

The necessary measures are represented by:

avoiding milk and dairy products;

avoiding products with gluten, i.e. all products that come from wheat, barley or rye;

identifying the foods that cause symptoms, as follows: consume a maximum of 3 foods per meal. If the symptoms appear, then one of the 3 foods is consumed one at a time and it is seen which ones produce the symptoms, in order to avoid them in the future. Repeat until all the respective foods are identified.

One of the causes of irritable bowel syndrome is the incomplete digestion of proteins in the stomach. Incompletely digested proteins reach the colon, where it irritates its mucosa, with the appearance of symptoms. The incomplete digestion of proteins occurs, as I said in the section on gastro-oesophageal reflux, due to the decrease in the acidity of the gastric juice, where I also indicate the treatment.

Ulcer

The most common cause of ulcers, both gastric and duodenal, is represented by Helicobacter pylori infection. This bacterium produces a substance that destroys the protective layer of the gastric and duodenal mucosa, thus favoring the appearance of ulcers.

There are studies that have shown that fresh cabbage juice is a very effective treatment for ulcers.

Thus, if you have an ulcer, prepare cabbage juice at home every day and drink 150 ml twice a day.

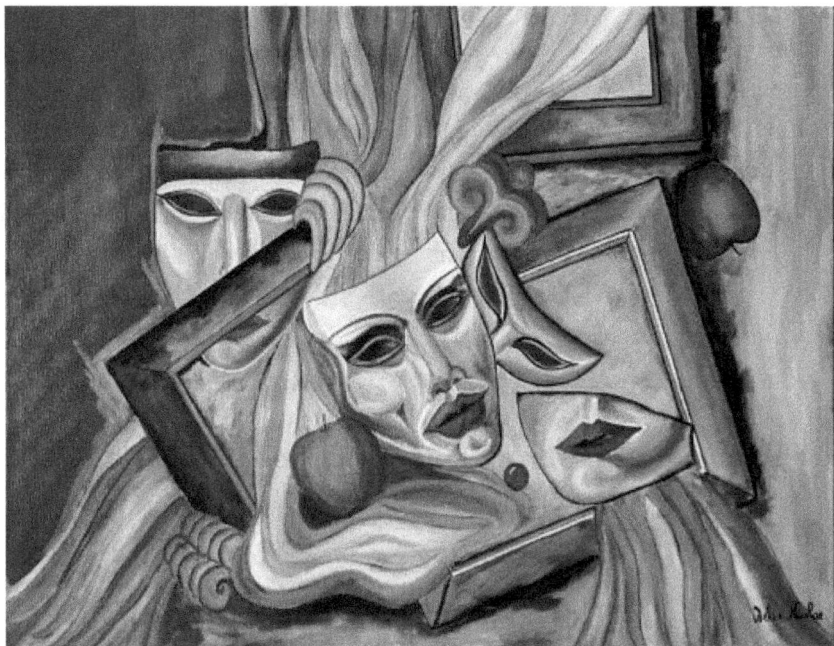

WEIGHT LOSS

In most cases, weight gain is caused by an increase in insulin secretion, which leads to insulin resistance. In this situation, insulin resistance must be reduced, which is achieved by low carbohydrate consumption and intermittent fasting. I detailed this topic in the "Lose weight easily with Doctor Cip" course.

To speed up the decrease in insulin resistance and speed up the weight loss process, you can prepare one of the following 3 solutions:

Solution with ginger, lemon, apple cider vinegar and cinnamon

ATTENTION: IT SHOULD NOT BE USED BY PEOPLE WITH GASTRITIS, ULCERS (BECAUSE APPLE VINEGAR INCREASES GASTRIC ACIDITY) OR BY PEOPLE TAKING BLOOD-THINNING TREATMENT (ANTICOAGULANTS, ANTIAGGREGANTS), BECAUSE GINGER HAS THE EFFECT OF REDUCING COAGULATION.

IF YOU TAKE SUCH A TREATMENT, ASK YOUR DOCTOR OR READ THE LEAFLET TO SEE IF IT HAS ANTICOAGULANT OR ANTIPLATELET ACTION.

Ingredients

1. A medium root (4-5 cm) of ginger, cut into pieces;

2. Two lemons with untreated peel (found at the supermarket): squeeze the juice, which is set aside, and cut the peel into pieces;

3. Cinnamon: two teaspoons of powder or two sticks;

4. Apple vinegar: 4 tablespoons;

5. Water: 2 liters.

Preparation method

Boil water.

When it starts to boil, add the ginger, lemon peels and cinnamon.

From that moment, leave 15 minutes.

After the 15 minutes, strain, let it cool for around 30 minutes and then add the lemon juice and apple vinegar.

Put the solution in a bottle, keep it in the fridge and drink 100-150 ml in the morning and in the evening before meals.

After taking the solution, do not eat for at least 15 minutes.

Drink the solution for 12 weeks. You can resume after a break of one month.

Solution with cucumber, ginger, lemon and mint

ATTENTION: IT SHOULD NOT BE USED BY PEOPLE WHO ARE TAKING TREATMENT THAT THINS THE BLOOD (ANTICOAGULANTS, ANTIAGGREGANTS), BECAUSE GINGER HAS THE EFFECT OF DECREASING COAGULATION.

IF YOU TAKE SUCH A TREATMENT, ASK YOUR DOCTOR OR READ THE LEAFLET TO SEE IF IT HAS ANTICOAGULANT OR ANTIPLATELET ACTION.

Ingredients and preparation method

1. Prepare the cucumbers:

- put 2 tablespoons of baking soda in 200 ml of warm water and mix well;

- add the peeled cucumbers, which you wash well in this solution;

- let it act for 15 minutes: baking soda inactivates any pesticides or insecticides that may be found in the peel;

- take out the cucumbers, cut them into pieces and put them in the blender.

2. Take a medium ginger root (4-5 cm), clean it and cut it into pieces, which you put in the blender;

3. Squeeze the juice from a lemon and pour it into the blender, where you add a handful of mint leaves, dry or fresh;

4. Add 500 ml of water and mix in the blender very well;

5. Drink the juice throughout the day.

Solution with cucumber, lemon, mint and cinnamon

Ingredients

1. 3 cornichon cucumbers;

2. A handful of fresh mint;

3. A lemon, preferably with untreated peel;

4. 2 spoons of cinnamon powder or 4 sticks.

Preparation method

1. Put 2 liters of water in a pot in which you put mint;

2. Prepare the cucumbers and lemon, if the peel is treated:

- put 2 tablespoons of baking soda in 200 ml of warm water and mix well;

- add the peeled cucumbers, which you wash well in this solution;

- let it act for 15 minutes: baking soda inactivates any pesticides or insecticides that may be found in the peel;

- take out the cucumbers, cut them into pieces and put them in the pot of water.

3. Cut the lemon into slices and put it in the pot of water;

4. Add the cinnamon;

5. Start the fire and leave it for 7-8 minutes from the moment it starts to boil;

6. Strain;

7. Drink 150 ml one hour before meals.

Soleus Pushups

I present to you a simple maneuver, which you can do while you eat, so that the blood sugar does not increase or increases moderately (it depends on the food you eat and in what quantities), so that the secretion of insulin does not increase or to grow moderately.

A few explanations to understand the mechanism: normally, active muscles do not directly consume glucose from the blood to obtain energy. In the muscles there are stores of glycogen, which consists of chains of glucose molecules. When the muscle contracts, glycogen is broken down into glucose molecules, which are burned for energy. Due to this fact, physical exercises do not lower blood sugar.

There is one exception, discovered by Professor Mark Hamilton, from the University of Houston, Texas: the soleus muscle (located on the back of the calf) has no glycogen reserves and directly consumes glucose from the blood.

He imagined an exercise, the soleus push-ups, which, thanks to the specificity of this muscle, lowers blood sugar: sit down, keep your knees bent at 90 degrees, keep your feet on the floor and rhythmically raise and lower your heels.

This simple exercise significantly lowers blood sugar. That's why I recommend you do it when you sit at the table, when you sit on the couch, when you sit at the office, whenever you have the opportunity.

In addition, this exercise also intensifies the burning of fats, with a decrease in their blood level.

Of course, these exercises do not replace the reduced consumption of carbohydrates, that is, you should not understand that, by doing push-ups, you can eat sweets and other carbohydrates in any quantity.

Frozen and/or fried bread

Bread contains starch, a carbohydrate that is made up of chains of glucose molecules.

In the intestine, these chains are broken down into glucose molecules, which are absorbed, causing an increase in blood sugar and insulin secretion. In essence, this is the mechanism by which bread makes you fat, because insulin causes the accumulation of fat and prevents the burning of stored fat.

However, there are methods by which bread can only cause a moderate and slow increase in blood sugar and therefore insulin secretion. It has been observed that if the bread is frozen or fried, a large part of the starch is no longer absorbed into the blood, so that it does not produce a sharp and rapid increase in blood sugar and insulin secretion. The effect is maximum if the two methods are combined, i.e. the bread is frozen and then, before eating, it is fried.

Similarly, cooked potatoes produce less of a rise in blood sugar if, after cooking, they are cooled and then reheated.

Foods that decrease the absorption of carbohydrates

The only foods that do not increase blood sugar or insulin secretion and also decrease the absorption speed and the amount absorbed in the intestine of carbohydrates are vegetables, greens and fat.

Thus, blood sugar and insulin secretion increase more slowly and reach a moderate maximum value, as such, it helps to lose weight.

That is why it is recommended that, at least at one meal, every day, you eat a salad, in which you put extra virgin olive oil and apple vinegar (this contributes to maintaining a normal blood sugar level).

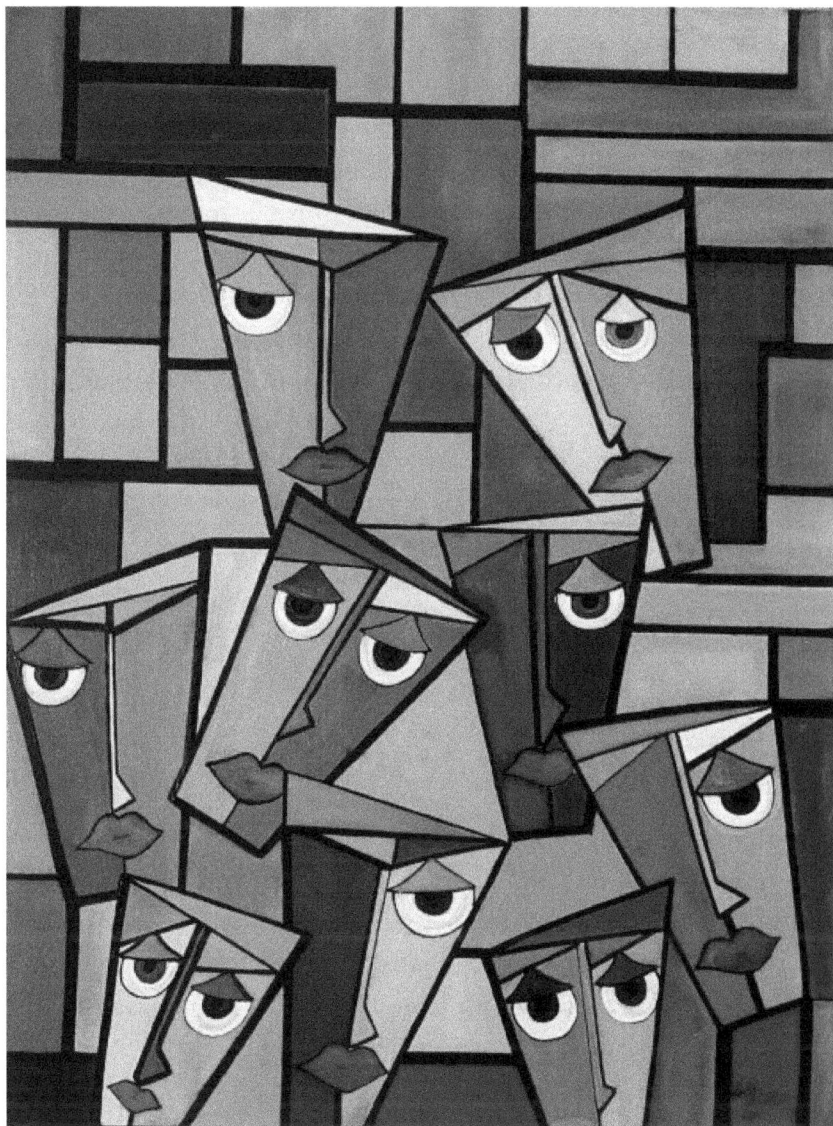

INTESTINAL PARASITOSES

Very often, intestinal parasites have non-specific manifestations: abdominal pain, diarrhea, constipation, hives.

If the cause of these manifestations is not found or the treatments have failed, it is possible to talk about a parasitosis.

In this case, you can try one of the following remedies:

1. wormwood tea;

2. garlic: as such (2-3 crushed cloves) or garlic capsules. If you take garlic as such, the cloves must be crushed and left in the air for 10-15 minutes, so that allicin, the active substance in garlic, becomes active;

3. American black walnut extract (tincture);

4. essential oil of cloves (caution, it must be diluted: 2 drops to a tablespoon of olive oil).

These products can be taken individually or combined.

NAUSEA

If you feel nauseous, for any reason, do a very effective acupressure maneuver: at the level of one forearm (it doesn't matter which one), identify, under the knuckle of the fist, the two tendons (they feel like two strings) and press with the thumb of the other hand in the space between them, 4-5 cm below the fist joint. Hold for 1-2 minutes and the feeling of nausea will disappear or decrease significantly.

STRESS

Stress is the body's coping and defense mechanism to various dangerous situations. Stress has a positive effect because it mobilizes the body's resources needed to respond to these situations.

However, prolonged stress has negative effects on health, affects the heart, causes increased blood pressure, depression, anxiety, insulin resistance with obesity and diabetes, decreased immunity, etc.

To reduce stress I recommend the following measures:

Eliminating the cause

Eliminating the cause is most effective, but very often impossible or very difficult.

So it is necessary to turn to other methods.

Avoiding news and talkshows

It is good to be informed, but not to sit in front of the TV for hours watching news or debates telling us that the apocalypse, economic crisis, global warming, drought, famine, cold and war are coming. Apart from the fact that they are presented in an alarmist manner, you can't change anything anyway and all you do is increase your stress levels.

It is preferable to watch entertainment shows, comedies, music, read something that relaxes you, take walks.

Lemon balm tea

70% of those who drink lemon balm tea report a decrease in stress, a state of calm and inner tranquility.

Walnuts

A study in Italy found that 50 grams of nuts a day reduced stress levels.

Fighting insomnia

Sleep and stress influence each other in the opposite direction: increased stress produces insomnia and poor quality, unrefreshing sleep, and insomnia and unrefreshing sleep increase stress.

Thus, it becomes mandatory to take the necessary measures to combat insomnia and get quality sleep.

To see what these measures are, see the next chapter.

INSOMNIA

To combat insomnia, to induce quality sleep, the following measures are possible:

Box breathing (breathing in square)

This is a technique developed by the US Navy SEALS, which reduces stress, calms and induces sleep.

The technique is very simple: breathe in for 4 seconds, hold for 4 seconds, breathe out for 4 seconds and hold for another 4 seconds. Repeat this cycle until you fall asleep, usually you won't exceed 10 cycles.

Sour cherry extract

Cherry extract has a sleep-inducing effect and combats insomnia.

Banana peel tea

Drink banana peel tea before bed in the evening. Be careful, bananas must have untreated peel. If you don't know whether it is treated or not, then, as a precaution, keep the banana for 15 minutes in a bicarbonate of soda solution (500 ml of water in which you put 2 tablespoons of bicarbonate of soda), then rinse it well under running water.

Nutmeg

Before going to bed, drink 100-150 ml of lukewarm milk in which you dissolve a teaspoon of nutmeg.

Chamomile tea

Before going to bed, smell a chamomile tea bag: it contains substances that stimulate the same area of the brain that is stimulated by benzodiazepines (a class of sedative drugs).

Sleeping with socks on

During sleep, the core temperature (inside the body) drops by about half a degree.

If you go to bed with socks on, the amount of blood reaching your feet increases and so more heat is lost through the skin, causing the core temperature to drop and the brain to be 'fooled' that you are already asleep and so enter the sleep state.

Lavender

Lavender contains substances that induce and maintain sleep.

The most effective form is essential oil, which can be used in this way:

1. by sniffing: put a few drops of essential oil on a towel or handkerchief close to your head or directly on your forehead;

2. orally: put one drop of essential oil in 2 liters of water and drink 100-150 ml before bedtime.

DEMENTIA

In Alzheimer's disease, a plaque formed by a material called amyloid forms around the neurons, which prevents glucose from entering the neurons, so they have no source of energy and slow down their functions, and some even die.

An alternative source of energy is ketone bodies, which are produced in the liver from fat and which pass through the amyloid plaque, enter neurons, which use them to produce energy. This partially increases neuronal activity and improves the symptoms of dementia.

A very good source of ketone bodies is coconut oil. It contains MCTs (medium chain triglycerides), which are converted in the liver into ketone bodies. You can also give MCT oil itself, which is extracted from coconut oil..

It has been observed that 3-4 weeks after taking coconut oil/MCT oil, the condition of the patient with dementia improves.

It should be noted that coconut oil does not cure dementia and taking it does not prevent dementia.

Take 2-3 teaspoons per day.

For the prevention of dementia, intermittent fasting appears to have a positive effect by lowering insulin resistance, which is a risk factor for dementia.

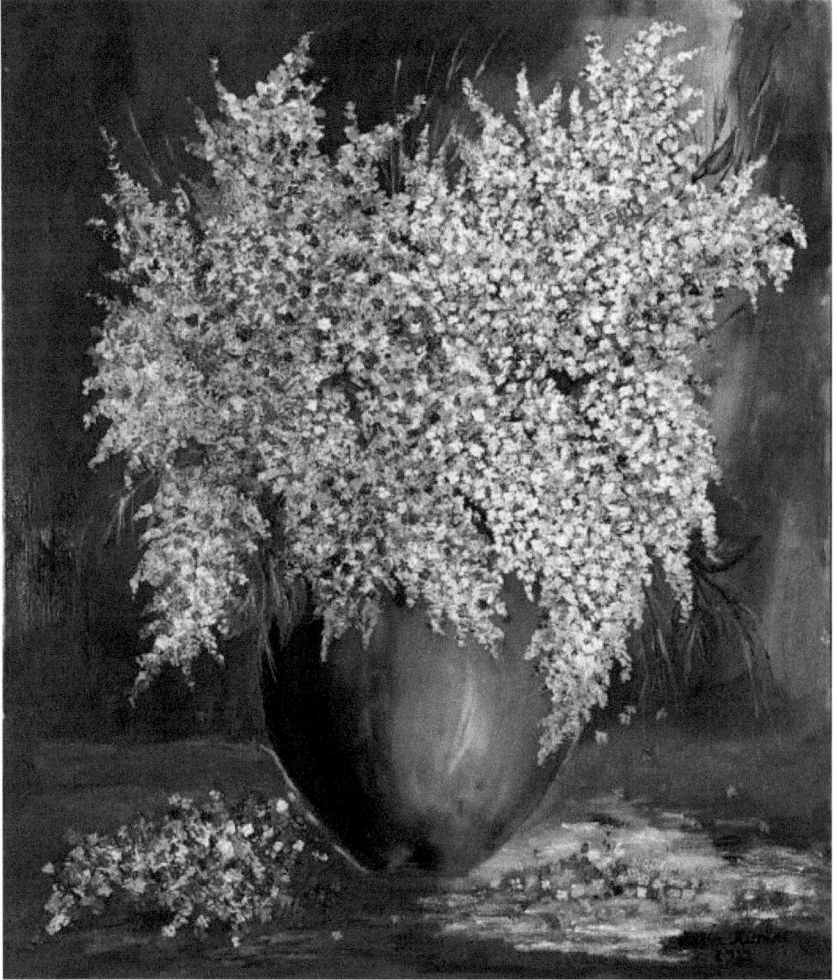

DEPRESSION

The following measures are useful in depression:

Sun exposure

Sunlight acts in depression by two mechanisms:

1. by increasing vitamin D synthesis. There are studies showing that depressed people have low vitamin D levels, and normalizing this can reduce depression;

2. by stimulating the retina, which increases the secretion of serotonin, a substance responsible, among other things, for mood (serotonin is also called the "happy hormone"). People with a normal level of serotonin are emotionally stable, calm and feel happy, while people with a low level are depressed and sad.

This explains why many depressions occur or worsen in winter or on cloudy days when the amount of light is reduced.

At times when there is not enough light, a 10,000 lux daylight lamp can be used for 30 minutes a day.

Stress reduction

Stress increases cortisol secretion, which causes a reduction in serotonin secretion.

For stress reduction, see the appropriate chapter.

Probiotics

In the gut, under the action of microbial flora, 95% of the body's serotonin is synthesized, among hundreds of other substances. An imbalance in the bacterial flora at this level often results in depression.

Warning: antibiotic abuse causes an imbalance of the intestinal microbial flora and can lead to depression.

Probiotic food supplements or probiotic foods such as sauerkraut, pickles or kefir, which contain a high amount of beneficial bacteria, can be given.

Intermittent fasting

Among many other health benefits, intermittent fasting also plays a role in reducing depression by increasing serotonin secretion and by its role in restoring the balance of gut microbial flora.

Vitamin D3

Studies on the efficacy of vitamin D3 administration are inconclusive, in that some have found an improvement in depression, others have not.

If there is a low level of vitamin D in the blood, it may be useful to take a vitamin D3 supplement at a dose of 10,000 IU per day, combined with 100 micrograms of vitamin K2 and 500 grams of magnesium.

Note: vitamin K2 is not involved in clotting, it is different from vitamin K1 (or vitamin K as it is commonly called), which is involved in clotting and is only available by prescription. Vitamin K2 is available without a prescription!

Vitamin D, because it needs a fatty environment to be absorbed, is taken with a meal or with a spoonful of olive oil.

PANIC ATTACK

In a panic attack, breathing becomes rapid, with short exhalation, leading to an exaggerated drop in the concentration of carbon dioxide in the blood, which in turn leads to the inability to use oxygen at the cellular level.

The following steps can be taken to stop panic attacks:

- Abdominal breathing, in which breathing movements are achieved solely by the movement of the diaphragm muscle, which moves up and down so that the abdomen inflates and deflates. Through these movements of the diaphragm, the parasympathetic nervous system is stimulated, which causes the calming down;

• breathing through the nose, inhaling for 4 seconds and exhaling for 4 seconds, which increases the concentration of carbon dioxide in the blood and increases oxygen utilization;

• bag breathing: breathing in and out in a bag increases the concentration of carbon dioxide.

VERTIGO

Vertigo is the sensation of spinning and can be one of two things: the person with vertigo has the sensation that they are spinning and things around them are standing still, or that they are standing still and things around them are spinning. In either case, the sensation is very unpleasant, accompanied by dizziness, loss of balance, nausea, vomiting.

Usually, vertigo is triggered by head movements.

One possible cause is calcium deposits in the inner ear.

It is therefore recommended to take vitamin D3, 10,000 IU per day, combined with 100 micrograms of vitamin K2 to remove these deposits.

(Note: vitamin K2 is not involved in clotting, it is different from vitamin K1 (or vitamin K as it is commonly called), which is involved in clotting and is only available by prescription. Vitamin K2 is dispensed without a prescription!)

Because vitamin D needs a fatty environment to be absorbed, it should be taken with a meal or with a tablespoon of olive oil, preferably extra virgin.

There are several maneuvers you can try to stop vertigo attacks:

1. sitting on a chair with handles, stand up, holding your hands on the handles, then bend forward with your head towards your knees, wait until the dizziness subsides and stay in this position for about 30 seconds. Then you suddenly sit back in the chair and stay there for another 30 seconds. If necessary, repeat the maneuver a few times;

2. massage in circular movements with your index finger at the point where the earlobe sticks to the head (it feels like a small indentation) for 30 seconds, then wait 1 minute, then repeat with the other ear. To prevent further attacks of vertigo, do this once a day.

TINNITUS

Tinnitus is that high-pitched, squeaky sound you hear in your ears that is not actually a real sound. It appears to be caused by a defect in the transmission of nerve impulses to the auditory nerve.

I present to you a maneuver invented by an American doctor, Dr. Jan Strydom, which is very effective, in many cases making the tinnitus disappear or at least significantly reduce.

Place the index finger over the middle finger on both hands, then bring your hands to the back of your head and snap your index fingers against the skull. Repeat these movements 10–20 times in a row. You can do 5–10 reps a day for up to 2 weeks.

After each round, assess the intensity of your tinnitus to see your progress.

In some people, the tinnitus disappears after 1-2 days, in others after a week to ten days, in others, fortunately few, it does not change.

LOSS OF SMELL AND/OR TASTE

If you've lost your smell and taste, you can try one of the two remedies below:

1. swallow a mixture of a teaspoon of turmeric, a tablespoon of olive oil and a teaspoon of ground pepper. Chances are that within a few dozen minutes your smell and taste will at least partially return. The effect is caused by the turmeric, and the olive oil and pepper are meant to increase the absorption of the turmeric.

(Turmeric is a spice, found in supermarkets.)

2. 9 ml of lavender syrup daily for 3-4 weeks.

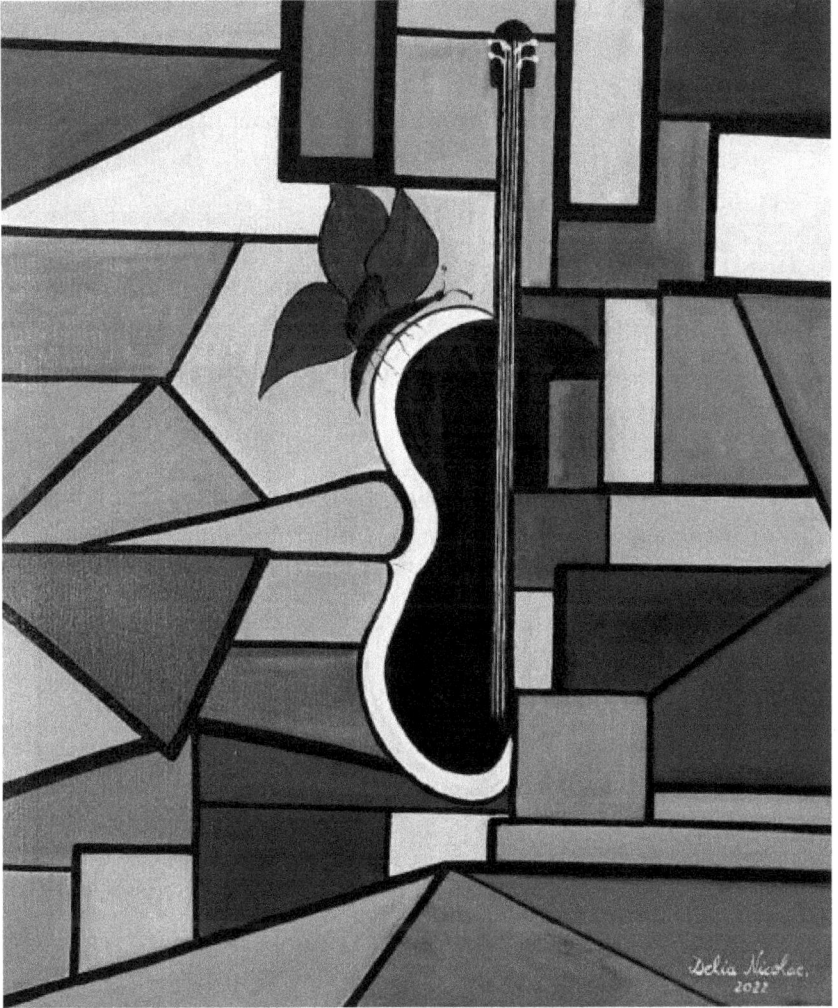

URINARY INFECTIONS

Urinary tract infections can be in the upper part of the urinary tract (pyelonephritis) or in the lower part (especially in the bladder, called cystitis).

Here are some natural herbal remedies with effective action:

Buchu, which is a plant native to South Africa, with antimicrobial, anti-adhesive (prevents microbes from adhering to mucous membranes) and diuretic action, thus favoring the destruction and elimination of bacteria through urine.

Cranberries, which have an anti-adhesive action (microbes cannot adhere to the urinary mucosa and are thus eliminated through urine).

Bearberries, which have antimicrobial and diuretic action.

Juniper, which has a very good antimicrobial action.

Oregano oil, which has a strong antibacterial effect. Note: take diluted, 1-2 drops in a tablespoon of olive oil.

Grapefruit seed extract, which has an antibacterial effect.

D-mannose, only for E. coli infections: prevents these bacteria from adhering to the urinary mucosa and thus being eliminated through the urine.

KIDNEY STONES

Here are 5 steps to avoid developing renal lithiasis (kidney stones):

1. drink at least 2 liters of water a day;

2. do not consume too much salt, as the sodium in salt increases calcium excretion through the urine, which increases the risk of developing stones;

3. most kidney stones are made up of calcium oxalate, which is produced by the combination of calcium and oxalic acid in the blood. To reduce the absorption of oxalic acid from the gut into the blood, eat foods with calcium, because calcium in the gut binds with oxalic acid, forming substances called oxalates, which are not absorbed into the blood.;

4. decrease consumption of foods high in oxalates (tea, chocolate, spinach, peanuts, beetroot, etc.);

5. In addition to calcium oxalate, kidney stones can also be formed from urates, substances that are produced from uric acid. Uric acid is formed in the body from fructose, so consumption of fructose should be limited and the main source of fructose is soft drinks and fruit juices, including fresh fruit juices. Therefore, avoid drinking juices of any kind.

AUTOIMMUNE DISEASES

Autoimmune diseases are those diseases in which the body secretes antibodies that attack its own structures, causing inflammatory damage to organs and tissues (skin, kidneys, blood vessels, joints, etc.).

Examples of autoimmune diseases: multiple sclerosis, rheumatoid arthritis, systemic lupus erythematosus, ankylosing spondylitis, atopic dermatitis (eczema), psoriasis, Hashimoto's thyroiditis.

The vast majority of people with autoimmune diseases have been found to have a vitamin D deficiency and/or an imbalance of microbial flora in the colon.

Thus, some general measures can be taken:

Vitamin D3 intake

It is recommended to take large doses, over 10,000 IU per day.

A Brazilian professor of neurology, Coimbra, has developed a protocol, which bears his name, in which very high doses of vitamin D3 are administered, going up to 120,000 IU per day. The dose is monitored by dosing parathormone (a hormone that plays a role in calcium metabolism). The results reported, as well as testimonials from patients treated with this protocol, are spectacular. Unfortunately, in Romania there are no doctors specialized in this protocol.

(Details here: https://www.coimbraprotocol.com/)

You can, however, try doses of up to 40,000 IU per day with monitoring of vitamin D blood levels: as long as this is below 100 ng/ml, vitamin D3 can be given without problems.

Vitamin D3 should be combined with vitamin K2 (preferably the MK7 version, which is the natural form of the vitamin), which prevents the deposition of calcium (whose absorption is stimulated by vitamin D) in organs and blood vessels and its deposition in bones. The dose is

100 micrograms per 10,000 IU of vitamin D3. There are preparations containing both vitamins in the appropriate doses.

(Note: vitamin K2 is not involved in clotting, it is different from vitamin K1 (or vitamin K as it is commonly called), which is involved in clotting and is only available by prescription. Vitamin K2 is dispensed without a prescription!)

Vitamin D3 should also be combined with magnesium, at a dose of 500 mg per day, as magnesium activates cell receptors for vitamin D.

Vitamin D3 needs fat to be absorbed, so it is advisable to take it with a meal or with a tablespoon of olive oil, preferably extra virgin.

Restoring the balance of intestinal microbial flora

This is done by eating probiotic foods (fermented foods such as kefir, sauerkraut and pickles) or probiotic supplements.

Intermittent fasting

It plays a role in restoring the balance of microbial flora and has an anti-inflammatory effect.

A special mention for **Hashimoto's thyroiditis**.

Normally gluten, which is the protein in wheat (so it is found in all flour, barley, rye products) is not absorbed in the gut. There is a condition of the gut, called 'coeliac disease', where gluten is absorbed into the bloodstream. As a foreign protein that has no place in the body, the body secretes anti-gluten antibodies, including anti-gliadin antibodies, as gliadin is a component of gluten. Gliadin has a chemical structure similar to a thyroid enzyme, so anti-gliadin antibodies attack the thyroid, causing Hashimoto's thyroiditis. So people with Hashimoto's thyroiditis should, in addition to other measures, stop eating gluten-containing foods.

ALOPECIA

If you have alopecia (baldness), a very effective remedy that causes hair growth is onion juice. A study was done using onion juice daily for 6 weeks, which resulted in hair growth on 83% of the hairless area in men and 73% in women.

The most effective is red onion juice.

Make a mixture of the juice of one onion, the juice of 2-3 cloves of garlic, a tablespoon of olive oil or coconut oil and 2-3 drops of rosemary oil, massage into the hairless areas and leave for at least 30 minutes (the longer the better). Repeat daily for 6 weeks.

If hair loss is on circular areas (on the head or on the chin in men), the condition is called "alopecia areata", which has an autoimmune cause, i.e. there are autoantibodies that attack the hair root.

In this situation, vitamin D3 can be given at a dose of 10,000 IU per day, combined with 100 micrograms of vitamin K2 and 500 mg of magnesium.

Vitamin D3 needs fat to be absorbed, so it is advisable to take it with a meal or with a tablespoon of extra virgin olive oil.

Note: vitamin K2 is not involved in clotting, it is different from vitamin K1 (or vitamin K as it is commonly called), which is involved in clotting and is only available by prescription. Vitamin K2 is available without a prescription!

HAIR LOSS

The cause of hair becoming brittle, falling out easily, can be vitamin deficiencies such as:

- vitamin C, which is corrected by eating vegetables and fruit;

- vitamin B7 (biotin), which is corrected by taking a biotin dietary supplement.

Other measures that can be taken to strengthen the hair are:

1. after washing your hair, rinse it with a solution of water and apple cider vinegar (3 tablespoons of apple cider vinegar to 1 liter of water), leave for 15 minutes and then rinse your hair with water;

2. apply shea butter to hair;

3. avoid shampoos with sulfates.

DANDRUFF

I recommend two solutions to get rid of dandruff:

1. after washing your hair, massage a mixture containing a tablespoon of linseed oil and 2-3 drops of oregano essential oil into your scalp and leave it on overnight. Repeat daily for a week. Dandruff will disappear for at least a while. If it recurs, repeat the treatment;

2. massage lavender oil into the scalp and leave for 48 hours. Repeat 3-4 times.

OILY HAIR AND SKIN

Hair and skin become greasy due to excessive secretion of sebum (the fatty substance secreted by the sebaceous glands, which are found in the skin), and this excessive secretion often occurs when the secretion of androgens (male hormones) is increased.

In women, androgens are secreted by the ovaries and adrenals.

The ovaries secrete too much androgen when insulin is elevated and the adrenals when stress levels are high.

The remedies are represented by:

1. stress reduction (see chapter on stress reduction);

2. reducing insulin levels by reducing carbohydrate intake (sugar products, flour, potatoes, rice) and intermittent fasting; for details, see the chapter on WEIGHT REDUCTION.

3. taking the DIM supplement, which has the effect of normalizing androgen levels.

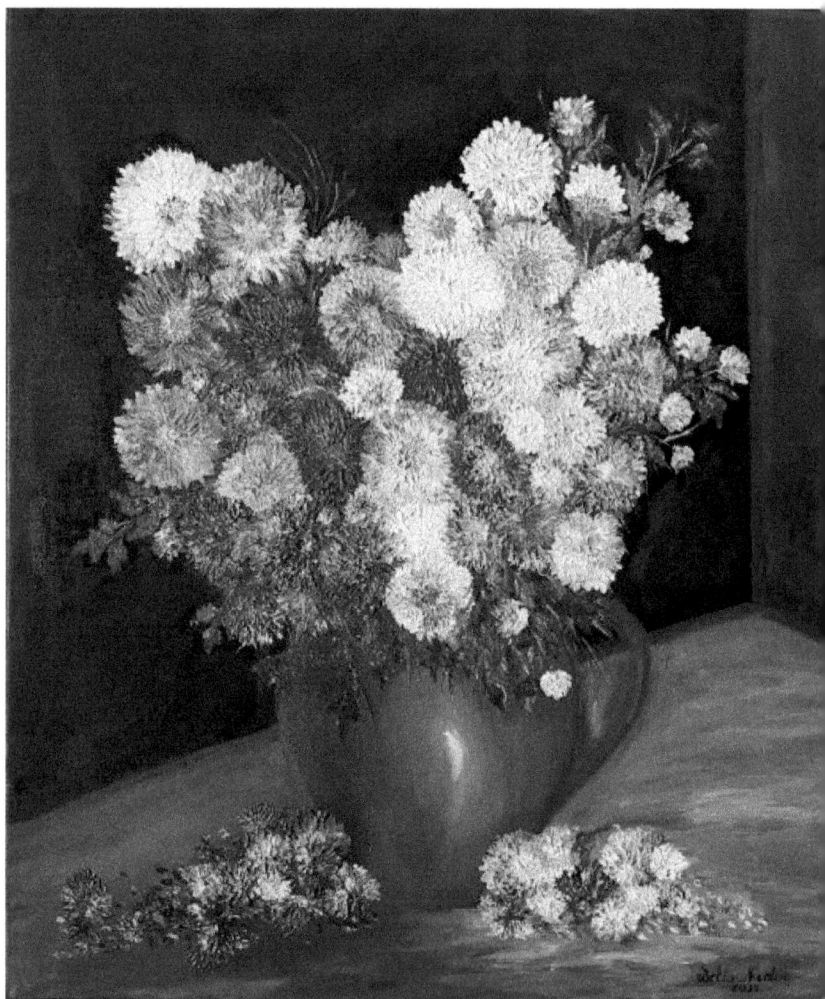

DRY SKIN

If you have dry skin, you can prepare a cream and apply it to your skin:

1. water: 6 teaspoons;

2. grinded chia seeds: 2 teaspoons;

3. seaweed powder: one teaspoon. Seaweed capsule powder can also be used;

4. a teaspoon of olive or coconut oil.

Mix well, apply to face or hands and leave on for 15 minutes.

Since dry skin is often caused by a deficiency of omega-3 fatty acids, it is good to eat foods rich in omega-3s (salmon, sardines, tuna, herring) or take them in the form of food supplements.

Bear in mind, however, that there may be other causes of dry skin: smoking, alcohol consumption, excessive consumption of sugar products, certain types of soap.

ACNE

Acne occurs at puberty and is caused by an excess of androgens (male sex hormones) which encourage the growth of bacteria on the skin and the production of plugs of dead skin cells that clog pores in the skin, leading to inflammation, redness and pain.

One of these bacteria secretes propionic acid, a substance that has a bad smell. That's why some teenagers have a bad smell, not because they don't wash.

Steps must be taken to restore androgen secretion to normal. Excessive increases in androgen secretion are caused by insulin and stress.

For stress reduction see that chapter.

To reduce insulin secretion, reduce consumption of sugary products, juices and eliminate snacks between meals (see chapter on WEIGHT REDUCTION).

Milk and dairy products, which have been found to cause acne through the androgens they contain, should also be reduced.

An effective supplement in reducing the effect of androgens is DIM. It is given 75-150 mg per day for up to 30 days. Effects may start to appear from the third or fourth day, but may occur later, and vary from case to case.

NAIL FUNGUS

The following is recommended for toenail fungus:

1. make sure your feet are dry and clean for as long as possible, as the fungus thrives in a damp environment;

2. apply a drop of tea tree essential oil or tincture of iodine to affected nails daily.

Note: the treatment is long lasting, on the order of weeks and even months, and requires patience and perseverance!

LOW HDL AND HIGH TRIGLYCERIDES

HDL is the form of cholesterol that protects the heart and blood vessels. Its concentration in the blood should not be below 40 mg/dl in men and below 50 mg/dl in women, but its protective action occurs at a value above 60 mg/dl.

If you have below 60 mg/dl, here are some steps you can take to raise your HDL:

1. intermittent fasting;

2. reduced consumption of sugar products, flour, potatoes, rice, fructose (no juices of any kind, not even fresh) and moderate consumption of fruit (favoring kiwi, strawberries, berries, plums, grapefruit);

3. avoiding alcohol;

4. consumption of saturated or monounsaturated fats: cold-pressed coconut oil, extra virgin olive oil, beef, salmon, herring, tuna, sardine, cod liver oil, butter;

5. avoiding polyunsaturated fats: sunflower oil, soybean oil, corn oil;

6. sleep between 7 and 9 hours;

7. quit smoking; if you can't, at least switch to vaping;

8. taking berberine in the first 1-2 months.

Triglycerides have a normal maximum blood concentration of 150 mg/dl. If it is higher, the risk of cardiovascular complications increases.

The following measures are useful to lower TG concentration:

1. intermittent fasting;

2. reduced consumption of sugar products, flour, potatoes, rice, fructose (no juices of any kind, including fresh fruit juices), moderate consumption of fruit, favoring kiwi, strawberries, berries, plums, grapefruit;

3. avoidance of alcohol;

4. replacing drugs that have the side effect of increasing TG: **talk to your doctor, don't do it yourself!!!**

GOUT

Gout occurs when the blood concentration of uric acid is increased. So preventing gout attacks is done by lowering uric acid levels.

Measures to reduce uric acid production

Reduced fructose consumption, because fructose in the body increases the secretion of substances called purines, from which uric acid is synthesized.

The most important source of fructose is carbonated or non-carbonated soft drinks (because they are sweetened with fructose-concentrated corn syrup), commercial 'no sugar added' natural juices (because they are made from fruit and have a high concentration of fructose) and fresh fruit juices, for the same reason, the high amount of fructose they contain.

So juices of any kind should be eliminated.

Measures to reduce uric acid concentration

The following supplements have the effect of lowering uric acid levels:

1. celery seed extract;
2. extract of black cherry;
3. zeolite.

Dosages are according to the package leaflet.

JOINT PAIN

If you have joint pain caused by joint inflammation (arthritis), here are two treatments.

Boron

Boron is the trade name for boron, which is a mineral with multiple effects in the body, including bone health. It has an anti-inflammatory effect on arthritis.

In a double-blind study conducted in 2009, the effect of boron administration in patients with arthritis was studied.

The study had two groups of patients, one group given boron and another group given placebo, a substance with no therapeutic effects. Patients had similar symptoms and were randomly assigned to the two groups. The study was double-blind, in the sense that neither patients nor doctors knew what was being given, boron or placebo.

The study lasted 14 days and each patient received 2 capsules per day.

The results showed that in half of the patients given boron, the effects were positive, compared to only 10% in the placebo group.

The dose is 6 mg per day.

Testimonial received on Tiktok:

"Doctor, I've been on Boron for 2 weeks and I feel excellent with a gonarthrosis I no longer feel."

Nettles

Another method of reducing joint pain is rubbing the joints with nettles. Nettles are effective in rheumatoid arthritis, arthritis and gout.

The exact mechanism by which nettles work is not known, but they significantly reduce inflammation and joint pain.

As you scrub, the stinging caused by the nettles will disappear. If necessary, use rubber gloves.

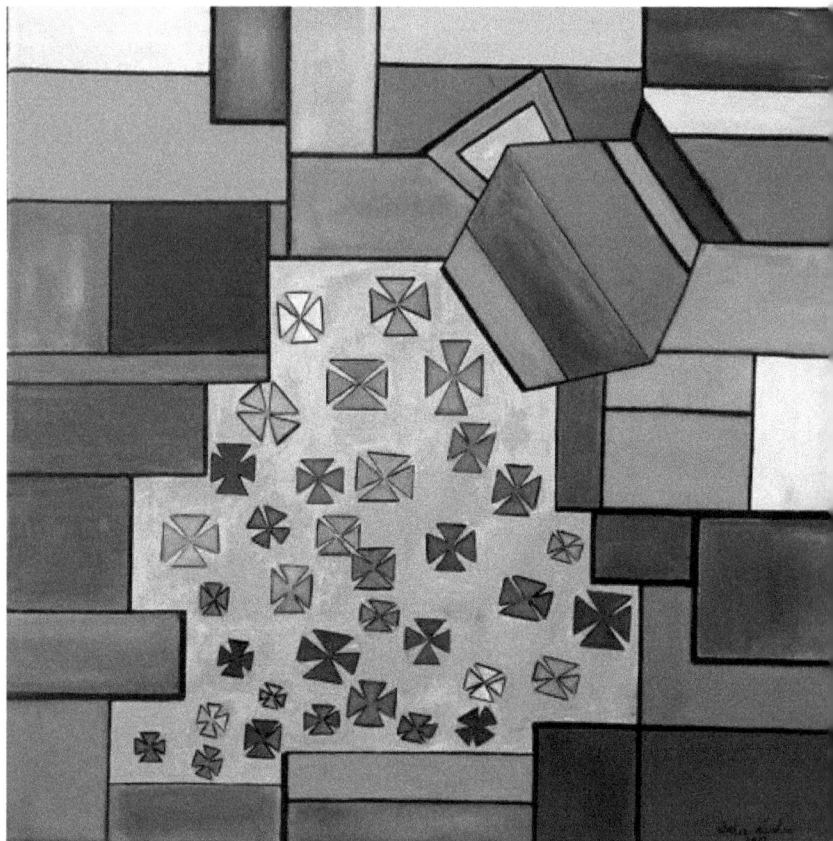

CANDIDIASIS

Candidiasis is the condition caused by candida. Candida is a fungus that is normally found in the body, on the skin, in the oral cavity, in the intestine, etc., but which does not manifest itself, is dormant and is kept in check by the beneficial bacterial flora.

In certain favorable situations, candida becomes active and candidiasis occurs, which is manifested by cravings for sweets, white tongue, itching in the vagina, anus, joint pain, fatigue, bloating, dermatitis, sinusitis.

Situations that cause candidiasis include an imbalance in the microbial flora (which occurs, for example, in prolonged treatment with antibiotics or in the consumption of milk and meat from factory-farmed animals that receive antibiotics in their feed and thus end up in our bodies), diabetes (candida develops in the presence of sugar), taking contraceptives, decreased immunity, stress, decreased gastric acidity (acid in the gastric juice destroys candida), treatment with gastric antacids.

The measures to be taken to combat candida are:

- intermittent fasting and reducing carbohydrate intake so that candida is deprived of food;

- restoring the balance of intestinal microbial flora by eating fermented foods (kefir, pickles, sour cabbage) or taking probiotics;

- taking oregano essential oil (dilute: 2 drops in a tablespoon of olive oil);

- eating garlic or garlic capsules;

- drinking an apple cider vinegar solution: one tablespoon of apple cider vinegar to 500 ml of water;

- coconut oil, which contains lauric acid, which has antifungal action.

CALLUSES

To prevent calluses, it is advisable not to wear shoes that are tight at the toe or espadrilles, as they have a flat and thin sole, creating increased pressure towards the front of the sole, favoring the appearance of calluses.

If you have calluses, you can try these two treatments:

1. keep the feet for 15-20 minutes in a basin of warm water in which you have dissolved 2-3 tablespoons of magnesium sulfate (it's called Epsom salt or bitter salt), then wipe them well and rub the corns gently with a pumice stone until the horny layer is removed. Then put Vaseline on the area and gently massage it into the skin.

Repeat every night until the calluses disappear.

2. massage the area of the calluses with sea buckthorn oil and within a week they may even disappear. This method even works on calluses between the fingers, where it is impossible to apply the first solution.

CONCLUSION

I hope you find these recommendations useful.

Please write me your feedback at doctorcip@doctorcip.eu.

Thank you!

Cheers!

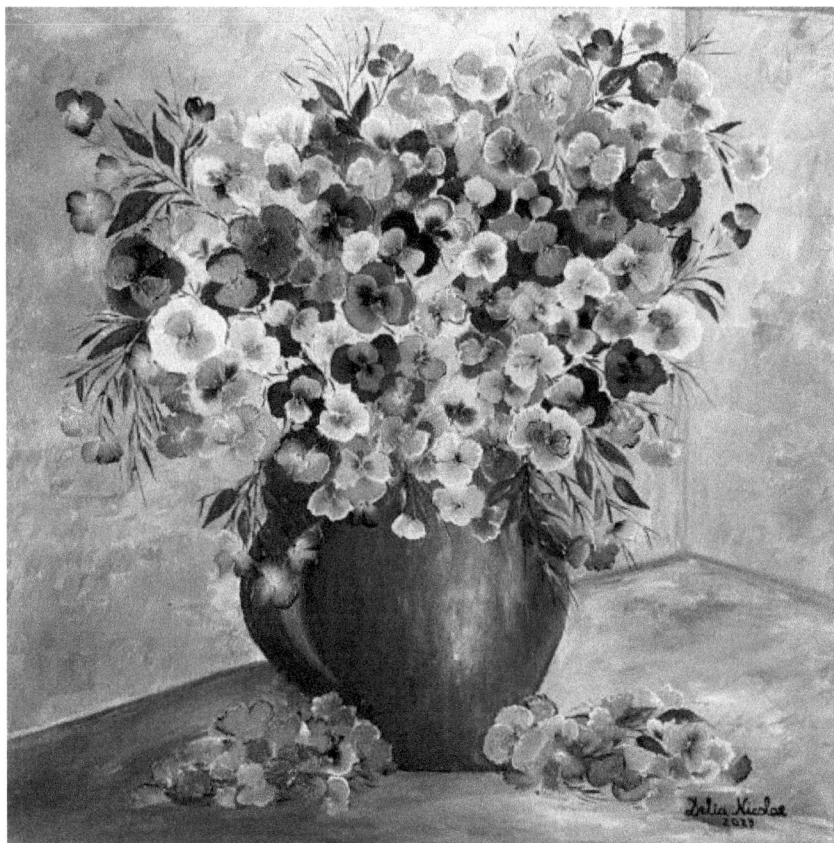

Ingram Content Group UK Ltd.
Milton Keynes UK
UKHW021950080523
421401UK00015B/938